I0703647

Thriving with Addison's Disease:

Making the Most of Life with a Chronic Illness

William Courson

ISBN-13: 979-8329206906

CONTENTS

CHAPTER 1: UNDERSTANDING ADDISON'S DISEASE

What is Addison's Disease?

Addison's disease, a disease I was diagnosed with in 2018, is a rare disease – it is estimated that it affects only about 0.05% of the population – that's about 4 out of every 100,000 persons. It was first described by a British physician Thomas Addison in 1855. Addison, for whom it is named, is a prominent figure in medical history and made several significant contributions to understanding various diseases, particularly in the realm of endocrinology (the study of the endocrine glands: the adrenals, the hypothalamus and the pineal gland, male and female gonads, pancreas, thymus, and the thyroid and parathyroid).

Thomas Addison was born in April 1793 in Longbenton, Northumberland, England. He studied medicine at the University of Edinburgh, where he earned his degree in 1815. Addison later joined Guy's Hospital in London, where he became a distinguished lecturer and physician. His keen interest in pathology and clinical medicine led him to explore diseases affecting the adrenal glands.

Addison's breakthrough came when he observed a group of patients exhibiting a distinct set of symptoms: chronic fatigue, muscle weakness, weight loss, low blood pressure, and skin hyperpigmentation.

Intrigued by these unclassifiable symptoms, Addison conducted meticulous autopsies and clinical examinations. He discovered that these patients had damaged adrenal glands, which he identified as the underlying cause of their symptoms.

His landmark paper, "*On the Constitutional and Local Effects of Disease of the Suprarenal Capsules*," published in 1855, detailed his findings and marked the first description of what would later be known as Addison's disease.

Addison's disease (also known as PAI or primary adrenal insufficiency) is an incurable and chronic condition that affects the adrenal glands, which produce (adrenaline, aldosterone, and cortisol) hormones that regulate a great many various bodily functions.

If you have been diagnosed with Addison's disease, you have damaged adrenal glands that are incapable of producing enough cortisol (and sometimes aldosterone) leading to a wide variety of symptoms that can on your daily life. Living with Addison's disease can be a challenge, as you must carefully manage your medication and monitor monitor your symptoms to prevent *adrenal crises*.

It is vitally important for those with Addison's to work closely with their healthcare tema (consisting at least of their primary health care provider and an endocrinologist) to develop a personalized treatment plan that meets their individual needs. This will include taking daily medication (such as corticosteroids) and being vigilant about recognizing the signs of an impending crisis.

Managing stress and anxiety is of critical concern if you have Addison's disease, as stress can quicky worsen symptoms and increase the risk of adrenal crises.

Techniques such as mindfulness meditation, deep breathing exercises, and regular physical activity can help reduce and eliminate needless stress and improve overall wellbeing. It is also important to prioritize self-care and seek support from loved ones or mental health professionals when needed.

Nutrition plays an absolutely central role in managing Addison's disease, as certain dietary measures can you're your support adrenal function and your overall health. Eating a balanced diet rich in fruits, vegetables, whole grains, and lean proteins can provide essential nutrients and energy. It is also important to stay hydrated and avoid excessive caffeine and alcohol which can negatively impact your adrenal function.

Exercising safely with Addison's disease is possible with the guidance of healthcare professionals and experienced trainers. Regular physical activity can help improve mood, reduce stress, and maintain a healthy weight.

It is critically important to listen to what your body is saying, start slowly, and gradually increase the intensity and duration of exercise. It is also crucial to monitor blood sugar levels and adjust medication as needed to prevent complications. A general rule of thumb is this: if it doesn't feel right, it isn't.

Causes and Symptoms of Addison's Disease

Addison's disease or PAI can occur when the adrenal glands don't produce enough of the hormones cortisol and aldosterone. The causes of Addison's disease can include:

Autoimmune Disorders: The most common cause, where the immune system attacks and destroys the adrenal cortex.

Infections: Chronic infections such as tuberculosis, HIV/AIDS, and certain fungal infections can damage the adrenal glands.

Adrenal Gland Disorders: Genetic disorders affecting adrenal gland development or function.

Cancer: Metastatic cancer that spreads to the adrenal glands.

Hemorrhage: Bleeding into the adrenal glands due to severe physical stress or injury.

Medications: Long-term use of corticosteroids, and certain antifungal and anticoagulant drugs, as well as cancer chemotherapy and immunotherapy drugs, can inhibit your adrenal function.

Surgery or Radiation: Removal of adrenal glands or radiation therapy targeting the adrenal area.

In my own case, which I'm informed is relatively rare (I know of only one other person, a woman in Namibia, Southwest Africa similarly affected) I developed PAI as a result of being treated for a metastatic skin cancer (melanoma) with two immunotherapy drugs, Opdivo (Nivolumab) and Yervoy (Ipilimumab), monoclonal antibodies which destroyed my adrenal glands along with the cancer.

My immune system was so potentiated by those drugs that it attacked not only the cancer cells, but every other part of my anatomy. My deranged immune response acted as though I were under massive assault by some infectious agent although I was not, and I went through all of the stages of sepsis and toxic shock syndrome (without there being any actual infection)

Any one or more of these factors may lead to the insufficient production of vital hormones, resulting in the symptoms associated with Addison's disease.

Symptoms of Addison's Disease can vary from person to

person in intensity and in its specific symptoms and signs but common ones include fatigue (which can sometimes be severe), weakness, weight loss (occasionally, weight gain), low blood pressure (occasionally high blood pressure), lower back pain, insomnia and darkening of the skin.

For many of the people affected, the most experienced symptom of Addison's Disease is fatigue, which can be debilitating. This fatigue is often accompanied by weakness and muscle aches, making it difficult to perform daily activities.

Other symptoms such as weight loss, nausea, and vomiting can also impact the quality of life for those with Addison's Disease.

It is important for everyone to be aware of these symptoms and seek medical attention if they experience them.

Addison's Disease is *Not* Adrenal Exhaustion

We hear a lot of talk these days of *Adrenal Exhaustion*. Addison's disease and adrenal exhaustion are two conditions related to adrenal gland function, but they differ enormously in terms of their causes, definitions, and medical recognition.

As we have discussed, Addison's disease, also known as primary adrenal insufficiency, is a rare but serious disorder where the adrenal glands do not produce enough of certain hormones, particularly cortisol and aldosterone. Addison's disease is typically caused by direct damage to or destruction of the adrenal glands. It is a recognized and accepted medical diagnosis.

Adrenal exhaustion, often referred to as adrenal fatigue, is a term used in alternative medicine to describe a collection of nonspecific symptoms that some believe are caused by chronic stress and resulting prolonged overuse of the adrenal glands.

This overuse is seen as resulting from prolonged physical or psychological stress, inadequate diet, lack of sleep, or physical or emotional trauma.

Adrenal exhaustion is not recognized by conventional medicine and lacks standardized diagnostic criteria. Alternative practitioners may use saliva cortisol tests or questionnaires.

While both conditions involve fatigue, Addison's disease has specific and severe symptoms related to hormone deficiencies. Adrenal exhaustion symptoms are more generalized and can overlap with many other conditions.
Understanding these distinctions is crucial for proper diagnosis and treatment. If someone suspects they have adrenal issues, it is important to consult a healthcare professional for accurate diagnosis and appropriate management.

"Adrenal Fatigue" can surely make you uncomfortable, but Addison's disease can kill you if you ignore it.

Diagnosis & Treatment Options

When it comes to actually living with Addison's disease, understanding the diagnosis and treatment options available to you is crucial. As I have said, Addison's disease is a rare condition that affects the adrenal glands, leading to a deficiency in cortisol and sometimes also aldosterone production.

Because Addison's is a rare disease affecting no more than around 10 out of every 100,000, one should be seen initially by an endocrinologist with experience in diagnosing and treating Addison's. Such a physician can be found by consulting one of the organizations listed in the "Resources" section at the end of this book.

Diagnosis typically involves blood tests to measure hormone levels and an ACTH stimulation test to assess adrenal function. Once diagnosed, treatment most likely involves hormone replacement therapy to replace the deficient cortisol and aldosterone.

Drug treatment may involve one or more of several options, including prednisone, prednisolone, hydrocortisone, and fludrocortisone, which are taken in tablet form, usually daily. Managing stress and anxiety with Addison's can be challenging, as stress can worsen your symptoms and if severe or prolonged can lead to adrenal crises. It's important to find healthy ways of coping such as mindfulness meditation, yoga, or psychotherapy to help manage stress levels. Additionally, ensuring you have a strong support system in place can be beneficial in times of heightened stress or anxiety.

Balancing work and social life with Addison's can be challenging but with proper planning and communication, it is achievable. Be open with your employer about your condition and any accommodations you may need. Additionally, maintaining a healthy work-life balance and setting boundaries can help prevent burnout and stress. Remember, it's okay to ask for help and prioritize self-care in order to thrive with Addison's disease.

Complications of Addison's Disease

Addison's can lead to a variety of complications and increase the risk of other health issues. Here are some conditions and complications that can:

Autoimmune Disorders:
Addison's disease is often caused by autoimmune adrenalitis, where the body's immune system attacks the adrenal glands. Individuals with Addison's disease are at higher risk for other autoimmune disorders, such as:
* Hashimoto's thyroiditis
* Graves' disease
* Type 1 diabetes
* Vitiligo
* Pernicious anemia
 *Celiac disease
* Primary Hypothyroidism
* Non-Toxic Goiter
* Coeliac disease
Infections:
People with Addison's disease are more susceptible to infections because cortisol plays a crucial role in the immune response. Common infections include:
* Tuberculosis (TB), which historically was a leading cause of Addison's disease
* Fungal infections
* Opportunistic infections, especially if the immune system is compromised

Adrenal Crisis:
This is a life-threatening emergency that can occur if Addison's disease is not adequately managed, characterized by:
* Severe weakness
* Low blood pressure
* Confusion or unconsciousness
* Electrolyte imbalances (e.g., hyperkalemia and/or

hyponatremia)
* Hypoglycemia: Insufficient cortisol production can lead to low blood sugar levels, causing symptoms such as dizziness, confusion, and in severe cases, loss of consciousness.

Bone Health Issues:
Chronic glucocorticoid therapy, often necessary to manage Addison's disease, can lead to:
*Osteoporosis
* Increased risk of fractures

Mental Health Issues:
Chronic illness and hormone imbalances can contribute to:
* Depression
* Anxiety
* Cognitive impairments

Cardiovascular Problems:
Low levels of aldosterone can lead to low blood pressure and electrolyte imbalances, affecting heart function and increasing the risk of cardiovascular disease.

Managing Addison's disease typically involves hormone replacement therapy to normalize cortisol and aldosterone levels, along with regular monitoring for potential complications and associated conditions. Early diagnosis and proper treatment are crucial to minimize the risk of additional health problems.

CHAPTER 2: LIVING WITH ADDISON'S

Adapting to Life with a Chronic Illness

Make no mistake: Addison's can kill you. And unless it is intelligently managed, it will kill you. There's a saying "All work and no play make Jack a dull boy." If Jack is an Addison's sufferer, his lack of sufficient downtime will make him a very sick boy.

Living with a chronic illness such as Addison's disease can be challenging, but with the right mindset and support, it is possible to thrive and live well. Adapting to life with Addison's requires a shift in perspective and a commitment to self-care. It is important to acknowledge the limitations imposed by the illness while also recognizing the many ways in which life can still be fulfilling and enjoyable.

Managing stress and anxiety is crucial for individuals with Addison's disease, as stress can exacerbate symptoms and lead to adrenal crises. Techniques such as mindfulness, deep breathing, and gentle exercise can help to reduce stress levels and promote a sense of calm. It is also important to prioritize self-care and make time for activities that bring joy and relaxation.

Nutrition plays a key role in managing Addison's disease, as certain foods can affect cortisol levels and overall health. It is important to maintain a balanced diet rich in fruits, vegetables, whole grains, and lean proteins. Avoiding processed foods, sugar, and caffeine can help to stabilize blood sugar levels and support adrenal function.

Consulting with a registered dietitian can provide personalized guidance on nutrition and dietary considerations for individuals with Addison's. If the person is being treated with steroids (which is likely) it is necessary to consume a diet adequate in calcium and sodium (but not too much sodium).

Exercising safely with Addison's disease is possible with careful planning and monitoring. Low-impact activities such as walking, yoga, and swimming can help to improve strength, flexibility, and overall well-being. It is important to listen to your body and adjust your exercise routine as needed to prevent fatigue and avoid triggering adrenal crises. Consulting with a healthcare provider before starting a new exercise program is recommended to ensure safety and effectiveness.

Balancing work and social life with Addison's disease can be challenging, but with the right support and accommodations, it is possible to thrive in both areas. Communicating openly with your employer about your condition and any limitations you may have can help to create a more supportive work environment. Prioritizing self-care and setting boundaries with social activities can help to prevent burnout and maintain a healthy balance in your life. Seeking support from friends, family, and healthcare providers can provide the encouragement and resources needed to navigate the challenges of living with Addison's disease.

Building a Support System

The saying goes *"You've got to have friends!"* and building a support system is essential for individuals who have been diagnosed with Addison's disease. This chronic illness can be challenging to manage on a daily basis, and having a strong support system in place can make a significant difference in your overall well-being. Whether it's friends, family, healthcare providers, or support groups, having people to turn to for help and guidance can provide much-needed comfort and reassurance.

Living with Addison's can be a daunting task, but with the right support system in place, it can become more manageable. Surround yourself with people who understand your condition and are willing to provide emotional support, practical assistance, and encouragement when you need it most. By building a network of individuals who can help you navigate the ups and downs of living with Addison's, you can feel more empowered and in control of your health.

Managing stress and anxiety is crucial for individuals with Addison's disease, as stress can exacerbate symptoms and lead to adrenal crises. Having a support system that includes mental health professionals, therapists, or support groups can help you develop coping strategies and techniques to manage stress effectively. By prioritizing self-care and seeking support when needed, you can better navigate the emotional challenges that come with managing a chronic illness like Addison's.

Nutrition and dietary considerations play a significant role in managing Addison's disease, and having a supportive network of healthcare providers, nutritionists, and peers can help you make informed choices about your diet. Your support system can offer guidance on meal planning, dietary restrictions, and nutritional supplements that can help you maintain optimal health and energy levels. By working with a team of experts and leaning on your support system for advice, you can ensure that your dietary needs are being met while managing Addison's disease effectively.

Building a support system is not just about managing your physical health – it's also about maintaining a balanced and fulfilling life. Whether it's finding ways to exercise safely, balancing work and social commitments, or navigating relationships and dating, having a support system in place can provide you with the tools and resources you need to thrive with Addison's disease. By reaching out to others for help and guidance, you can create a strong foundation for living well with a chronic illness and ensure that you have the support you need to thrive in all areas of your life.

Setting Realistic Expectations

Every one of us, especially those dealing with a chronic debilitating disease, needs to ask themselves how much is one capable of in terms of daily exertion. All human beings are born as equals, but we are not all born identical. Every single one of us has some "weak link" in our chain, and setting realistic expectations is a crucial aspect of managing Addison's disease. It is important for individuals who have been diagnosed with this chronic illness to understand that their health may fluctuate and that they may experience periods of fatigue, weakness, and other symptoms.

By setting realistic expectations for themselves, individuals can better cope with the challenges of living with Addison's and take proactive steps to manage their health effectively.

When setting realistic expectations, it is important for individuals with Addison's to recognize their limitations and prioritize self-care. This may involve making adjustments to their daily routine, such as getting adequate rest, eating a balanced diet, and taking medications as prescribed. By acknowledging their limitations and taking steps to care for themselves, individuals can better manage their symptoms and prevent adrenal crises. Managing stress and anxiety is also essential for individuals with Addison's disease.

Stress can exacerbate symptoms and lead to adrenal crises, so it is important for individuals to find healthy ways to cope with stress and anxiety. This may involve practicing relaxation techniques, such as deep breathing or meditation, engaging in regular exercise, or seeking support from a therapist or support group.

Nutrition and dietary considerations are important for individuals with Addison's disease. It is important for individuals to maintain a balanced diet that includes plenty of fruits, vegetables, whole grains, and lean proteins. It is also important for individuals with Addison's to stay hydrated and avoid excessive consumption of caffeine, alcohol, and sugary foods, which can exacerbate symptoms and lead to adrenal crises.

In conclusion, setting realistic expectations is essential for individuals with Addison's disease to effectively manage their health and well-being. By acknowledging their limitations, prioritizing self-care, managing stress and anxiety, and maintaining a healthy diet, individuals can better cope with the challenges of living with Addison's. It is important for individuals with Addison's to seek support from healthcare providers, therapists, and support groups to help them navigate the complexities of living with a chronic illness and find ways to thrive despite their diagnosis.

CHAPTER 3: MANAGING STRESS AND ANXIETY WITH ADDISON'S

The Impact of Stress on Addison's Disease

Stress can make anyone a mess, but if that person has Addison's it can do much more than simply make a mess of oneself. Stress can have an extremely significant impact on individuals living with Addison's disease. This chronic illness affects the adrenal glands, which are responsible for producing essential hormones like cortisol and aldosterone. When stress levels are high, the adrenal glands may struggle to keep up with the body's demands, leading to a potential exacerbation of Addison's symptoms. It is crucial for individuals with Addison's to manage stress effectively in order to maintain their overall health and well-being.

Managing stress and anxiety is essential for those with Addison's disease. Techniques such as deep breathing, meditation, and mindfulness can help to reduce stress levels and promote relaxation. It is also important to establish a support system of friends, family, and healthcare providers who can provide emotional support during times of stress. Additionally, engaging in activities that bring joy and relaxation, such as hobbies or spending time in nature, can help to alleviate stress and improve overall quality of life.

Nutrition plays a crucial role in managing Addison's disease and reducing the impact of stress on the body. Eating a balanced diet rich in fruits, vegetables, whole grains, and lean proteins can help to support adrenal function and overall health. It is important for individuals with Addison's to monitor their sodium intake, as low levels of aldosterone can lead to salt cravings. Working with a registered dietitian can help individuals with Addison's to develop a personalized nutrition plan that meets their unique needs.

Exercise is an important component of managing Addison's disease, but it is essential to do so safely. Individuals with Addison's should consult with their healthcare provider before starting a new exercise routine to ensure that it is safe for their condition. Low-impact activities like walking, swimming, or yoga can help to reduce stress levels and improve overall health. It is important to listen to your body and adjust your exercise routine as needed to prevent overexertion.

Finding a balance between work, social life, and self-care is key for individuals living with Addison's disease. It is important to prioritize self-care activities like getting enough rest, eating well, and managing stress in order to maintain overall health. Building a strong support system of friends, family, and healthcare providers can also help individuals with Addison's to navigate the challenges of living with a chronic illness. By taking a proactive approach to managing stress and prioritizing self-care, individuals with Addison's can thrive and live well with their condition.

Stress-Relief Techniques and Coping Strategies

Living with Addison's disease can bring about a unique set of challenges, including managing stress and anxiety. It's important for individuals with Addison's to develop stress- relief techniques and coping strategies to help them navigate the ups and downs of living with a chronic illness. One very effective way to reduce stress and anxiety is through mindfulness and relaxation techniques such as deep breathing exercises, meditation, and yoga. These practices can help calm the mind and body, allowing individuals to better cope with the daily stresses of managing Addison's.

Nutrition and dietary considerations play a crucial role in

managing Addison's disease. It's important for individuals with Addison's to follow a well-balanced diet that includes plenty of fruits, vegetables, whole grains, and lean proteins. Avoiding processed foods, sugary snacks, and caffeine can also help regulate blood sugar levels and prevent adrenal fatigue. Consulting with a registered dietitian who specializes in Addison's disease can provide personalized guidance on nutrition and dietary choices to support overall health and well-being.

Exercising safely with Addison's disease is possible with careful planning and monitoring. It's important for individuals with Addison's to listen to their bodies and not push themselves too hard during workouts. Engaging in low-impact activities such as walking, swimming, or gentle yoga can help improve strength, flexibility, and overall well-being. Staying hydrated and monitoring blood sugar levels before, during, and after exercise is also important to prevent adrenal crises and promote optimal health

Balancing work and social life with Addison's disease can be challenging, but with the right strategies in place, it is possible to thrive in both areas. Setting boundaries, prioritizing self-care, and communicating openly with colleagues and friends about your condition can help reduce stress and promote a healthy work-life balance. Seeking support from coworkers, friends, and family members can also provide valuable emotional support and encouragement during times of need.

In conclusion, developing stress-relief techniques and coping strategies, focusing on nutrition and dietary considerations, exercising safely, and balancing work and social life are essential components of living well with Addison's disease.

By taking a proactive approach to managing stress, staying

mindful dietary choices, engaging in safe exercise, and fostering healthy relationships and support systems, individuals with Addison's can thrive and lead fulfilling lives despite the challenges of living with a chronic illness.

Seeking Professional Help for Anxiety

Dealing with anxiety is a relatively frequent experience for many individuals living with Addison's disease. The constant management of medication, stress, and potential adrenal crises can contribute to heightened feelings of anxiety. Seeking professional help for anxiety is an important step in managing your mental health and overall well-being. A mental health professional, such as a therapist or counselor, can provide valuable support and guidance in coping with anxiety and developing healthy coping mechanisms.

When seeking professional help for anxiety, it is important to find a therapist or counselor who has experience working with individuals living with chronic illnesses, such as Addison's disease. They will have a better understanding of the unique challenges and stressors that come with managing a chronic illness and can provide tailored support and strategies to help you cope with anxiety effectively. Additionally, they can help you navigate the emotional impact of living with a chronic illness and develop resilience in the face of adversity.

Therapy can provide a safe space for you to explore and process your feelings of anxiety, as well as any other emotional challenges you may be facing. Through therapy, you can learn effective coping skills, relaxation techniques, and mindfulness practices to manage anxiety symptoms and reduce stress. Your therapist can also help you identify and challenge negative thought patterns and beliefs that may be contributing to your anxiety, and support you in developing a more positive and resilient mindset.

In addition to therapy, medication may also be recommended to help manage anxiety symptoms. It is important to work closely with your healthcare provider to find the right medication and dosage that works best for you. Some individuals with Addison's disease may need to be cautious when taking certain medications, as they can interact with their adrenal hormone replacement therapy. Your healthcare provider can help you navigate these considerations and ensure that your treatment plan is safe and effective.

Remember, seeking professional help for anxiety is a proactive step in taking care of your mental health and well-being. You are not alone in your struggles, and there are resources and support available to help you manage anxiety and thrive with Addison's disease. Don't hesitate to reach out for help and prioritize your mental health – you deserve to live a fulfilling and balanced life, even with a chronic illness.

CHAPTER 4: NUTRITION AND DIETARY CONCERNS FOR THOSE WITH ADDISON'S

Importance of a Balanced Diet

When I developed Addison's, I very quickly noticed that my appetite had changed: unlike many Addison's patients I did not lose my appetite, I still very much enjoyed food. However, I found myself incapable of eating it in three large (or large-ish) meals daily. I found it necessary to consume five or six smaller meals throughout the day, and this greatly increased my comfort level with food. I suspect other Addison's sufferers may have the same experience.

A balanced diet is crucial for individuals with Addison's disease as it plays a significant role in managing symptoms and promoting overall health. People diagnosed with Addison's need to pay close attention to their nutrition and dietary choices to ensure they are getting the necessary nutrients to support their adrenal function. A balanced diet can help regulate blood sugar levels, maintain energy levels, and support the immune system, all of which are essential for managing Addison's disease effectively.

It is important for individuals with Addison's to focus on eating a variety of nutrient-dense foods such as fruits, vegetables, whole grains, lean proteins, and healthy fats. These foods provide essential vitamins, minerals, and antioxidants that can help support adrenal function and overall well-being.

It is also important to avoid processed foods, sugary snacks, and high-fat foods, as they can contribute to inflammation, weight gain, and other health issues that can exacerbate symptoms of Addison's disease.

In addition to making healthy food choices, individuals with

Addison's should also pay attention to their meal timing and portion sizes.

Eating regular meals and snacks throughout the day can help stabilize blood sugar levels and prevent energy crashes.

It is also important to listen to your body and eat when you are hungry, rather than waiting until you are extremely hungry, as this can lead to overeating and blood sugar imbalances.
It is recommended that individuals with Addison's work with a healthcare provider or registered dietitian to develop a personalized nutrition plan that meets their individual needs and supports their overall health.

A healthcare provider can help identify any nutrient deficiencies, food sensitivities, or other dietary issues that may be impacting adrenal function and provide guidance on how to address them through diet and supplementation.

By focusing on a balanced diet and making healthy food choices, individuals with Addison's can better manage their symptoms, improve their energy levels, and support their overall well-being. It is important to prioritize nutrition and dietary considerations as part of a holistic approach to managing Addison's disease and promoting a healthy lifestyle.

Foods to Avoid and Include

Living with Addison's disease can present unique challenges, especially when it comes to managing your diet. Certain foods can have a negative impact on your health and well-being, while others can provide essential nutrients to support your body. In this subchapter, we will explore the foods to avoid and include in your diet to help you thrive with Addison's disease.

When it comes to foods to avoid, it is important to steer clear of high-sodium processed foods. These can cause fluid retention and increase your blood pressure, which can be particularly dangerous for those with Addison's disease. Additionally, foods high in sugar and refined carbohydrates can lead to fluctuations in blood sugar levels, which can exacerbate symptoms of fatigue and weakness.

On the flip side, there are certain foods that can be beneficial for individuals with Addison's disease. Incorporating nutrient-dense foods such as fruits, vegetables, whole grains, lean proteins, and healthy fats can help support your overall health and well-being.

These foods provide essential vitamins, minerals, and antioxidants that can help boost your immune system and energy levels.

By way of summary:

Food to emphasize in your diet include:

Milk
Cheese (incl. Ricotta and Cottage)
Yogurt
Grain products
Soy Milk
Turnip Greens
Kale Broccoli
Tofu
Eggs
Cheese
Chicken
Soups
Canned Tuna

Fortified Cereals
Fortified Orange Juice
Canned Beans
Salted Nuts
Salted Seeds
Added Table Salt* (*speak with your physician if you have high blood pressure)

Food to remove from your diet include:

Salt Substitutes
Coffee
Geen Tea
Black Tea
Too much Alcohol
Too many Bananas
Too any Oranges

It is also important to pay attention to your fluid intake, as dehydration can be a common issue for those with Addison's disease. Drinking an adequate amount of water and avoiding excessive caffeine and alcohol can help prevent dehydration and support your body's ability to function optimally. The National Academy of Medicine (USA) suggests around 125 ounces per day for males, and 91 ounces for females.

In addition to focusing on the foods you eat, it is also important to consider how you eat. Eating regular, balanced meals and snacks throughout the day can help stabilize your blood sugar levels and provide a steady source of energy. Listening to your body's hunger and fullness cues can also help prevent overeating or undereating, both of which can impact your energy levels and overall health.

By being mindful of the foods you consume and making conscious choices to support your body's needs, you can better manage your symptoms and thrive with Addison's disease. Remember to work closely with your healthcare team to develop a personalized nutrition plan that meets your individual needs and supports your overall well-being.

Meal Planning and Nutritional Supplements

Meal planning and nutritional supplements are essential components of managing Addison's disease effectively. People with Addison's must pay close attention to their diets to ensure they are getting the nutrients they need to support their adrenal function. Planning meals ahead of time can help individuals with Addison's maintain stable blood sugar levels and avoid adrenal crises.

Nutritional supplements can also play a crucial role in supporting adrenal health. People with Addison's may benefit from taking supplements such as vitamin C, B vitamins, magnesium, and zinc to support their adrenal glands. It is important to consult with a healthcare provider or nutritionist before starting any new supplement regimen to ensure it is safe and appropriate for individual needs.

When meal planning for Addison's disease, it is important to focus on a balanced diet that includes a variety of nutrient-dense foods. This may include lean proteins, whole grains, fruits, vegetables, and healthy fats. Avoiding processed foods, excess sugar, and caffeine can also help support adrenal health and prevent spikes in blood sugar levels.

In addition to meal planning, individuals with Addison's should also pay attention to the timing of their meals and snacks. Eating smaller, more frequent meals throughout the day (as was the case with myself) can help maintain stable blood sugar levels and prevent energy crashes. It is also important to stay hydrated and drink plenty of water to support overall health and wellbeing.

Overall, meal planning and nutritional supplements are important tools for managing Addison's disease and supporting adrenal health. By focusing on a balanced diet, timing meals appropriately, and incorporating supplements as needed, individuals with Addison's can better manage their symptoms and live well with this chronic illness.

Consulting with healthcare providers and nutritionists can help individuals create a personalized meal plan that meets their unique needs and supports their overall health and wellbeing.

CHAPTER 5: EXERCISING SAFELY WITH ADDISON'S

Benefits of Exercise for Addison's Patients

For the better part of my life, I have been an enthusiastic couch potato, with very little interest in exercise. My Addison's diagnosis removed that "luxury" from my existence. For now, walking, swimming, yoga, and cycling are my favored forms of physical activity, but the opportunities for swimming and cycling are few and far between. Nonetheless, walking and yoga are excellent means for the Addison's patient to keep in shape.

Regular exercise is an essential component of managing Addison's disease, as it can provide numerous benefits to individuals living with this chronic illness. Engaging in physical activity can help improve overall health and well-being, as well as enhance energy levels and reduce feelings of fatigue. Exercise can also help to regulate blood sugar levels, improve cardiovascular health, and boost mood and mental clarity. By incorporating regular exercise into your routine, you can better manage your symptoms and improve your quality of life.

One of the key benefits of exercise for individuals with Addison's disease is its ability to help manage stress and anxiety. Regular physical activity has been shown to reduce feelings of stress and anxiety, as well as improve mood and mental well-being. By engaging in activities such as yoga, Pilates, or gentle aerobic exercise, individuals with Addison's can effectively manage their stress levels and improve their overall mental health. Exercise can also help to promote relaxation and improve sleep quality, which are important factors in managing stress and anxiety.

In addition to managing stress and anxiety, exercise can also play a crucial role in maintaining a healthy weight and managing blood sugar levels for individuals with Addison's disease. Regular physical activity can help to improve insulin sensitivity, which is important for individuals with Addison's who may experience fluctuations in blood sugar levels. By incorporating a combination of aerobic exercise, strength training, and flexibility exercises into your routine, you can better manage your weight and blood sugar levels, as well as improve your overall health and well-being.

It is important for individuals with Addison's disease to exercise safely and listen to their bodies during physical activity. It is recommended to start slowly and gradually increase the intensity and duration of your workouts. It is also important to stay hydrated, monitor your blood sugar levels, and take breaks as needed. Consult with your healthcare provider before starting any new exercise program to ensure that it is safe and appropriate for your individual needs and health status.

Overall, incorporating regular exercise into your routine can provide numerous benefits for individuals living with Addison's disease. From managing stress and anxiety to improving cardiovascular health and maintaining a healthy weight, exercise can play a crucial role in managing symptoms and improving quality of life. By finding activities that you enjoy and can safely engage in, you can reap the many benefits of exercise and thrive with Addison's disease.

Types of Exercise to Consider

When it comes to managing Addison's disease, incorporating regular exercise into your routine can be incredibly beneficial. However, it is important to choose the right types of exercise to ensure that you are not putting undue stress on your body. Some types of exercise to consider include low-impact activities such as walking, swimming, or gentle yoga. These types of exercise can help to improve your overall fitness level without putting too much strain on your adrenal glands.

Strength training is another important type of exercise to consider for those with Addison's disease. Building muscle can help to improve your overall strength and stamina, which can be especially important when dealing with a chronic illness. However, it is important to start slowly and gradually increase the intensity of your workouts to avoid overexerting yourself.

Working with a personal trainer who is knowledgeable about Addison's disease can also be helpful in creating a safe and effective strength training program.

Cardiovascular exercise is another important component of a well-rounded exercise routine for individuals with Addison's disease. Activities such as biking, jogging, or dancing can help to improve your heart health and overall cardiovascular fitness. However, it is important to listen to your body and stop if you start to feel fatigued or dizzy. It is also important to stay hydrated and monitor your blood sugar levels before, during, and after exercise to ensure that you are staying safe and healthy.

In addition to these types of exercise, it is also important to incorporate flexibility and balance training into your routine. Activities such as stretching, Pilates, or Tai Chi can help to improve your flexibility and balance, which can be important for preventing falls and injuries. These types of exercise can also help to reduce stress and improve your overall sense of well-being, which can be especially important when dealing with a chronic illness like Addison's disease.

Overall, the key to exercising safely with Addison's disease is to listen to your body, start slowly, and gradually increase the intensity of your workouts. It is also important to work with a healthcare provider or personal trainer who is knowledgeable about Addison's disease to ensure that you are exercising in a way that is safe and effective for your individual needs. By incorporating a variety of different types of exercise into your routine, you can improve your overall fitness level and quality of life while managing your Addison's disease effectively.

Precautions and Guidelines for Exercising

Exercising is an important aspect of maintaining overall health and well-being, especially for individuals with Addison's disease. However, there are certain precautions and guidelines that should be followed to ensure that exercise is done safely and effectively. In this subchapter, we will discuss some key considerations for exercising with Addison's disease.

First and foremost, it is crucial to consult with your healthcare provider before starting any exercise regimen. They can provide guidance on the types of exercises that are safe for you to do, as well as any modifications that may be necessary. It is also important to monitor your symptoms during exercise and adjust your routine accordingly.

When exercising with Addison's disease, it is important to listen to your body and not push yourself too hard. Pay attention to signs of fatigue, dizziness, or weakness, and take breaks as needed. It may also be helpful to keep a log of your workouts and symptoms to track your progress and identify any patterns or triggers.

In terms of specific types of exercise, low-impact activities

such as walking, swimming, or yoga are generally safe choices for individuals with Addison's disease. These types of exercises can help improve cardiovascular health, strength, and flexibility without putting too much stress on the body.
It is also important to stay hydrated and fuel your body properly before and after exercise. Make sure to drink plenty of water and eat a balanced meal or snack that includes carbohydrates and protein to support your energy levels and recovery. Additionally, be mindful of any medications you may be taking and how they may affect your exercise routine.

Exercising with Addison's disease can be a positive and beneficial experience when done safely and mindfully. By following these precautions and guidelines, you can enjoy the many physical and mental health benefits of regular exercise while managing your condition effectively.

CHAPTER 6: BALANCING WORK & SOCIAL LIFE WITH ADDISON'S

Communicating with Employers and Colleagues

It's key to let the important people in your life (employers, colleagues, friends, and others) know about your condition and the limitations that it may entail for them.

Communicating with employers and colleagues is an important aspect of managing Addison's disease in the workplace. It is crucial to educate your employer and colleagues about your condition to ensure a safe and supportive work environment. Be open and honest about your needs and limitations, and discuss any accommodations that may be necessary to help you thrive in your job.

When communicating with employers, it is important to emphasize the importance of flexibility and understanding. Let them know that while you may have limitations due to Addison's disease, you are still capable of performing your job duties with the right support. Discuss any potential triggers for adrenal crises and how they can be avoided in the workplace.

In addition to communicating with your employer, it is also essential to keep your colleagues informed about your condition. This can help create a supportive network of coworkers who understand your needs and can assist in case of an emergency. Consider sharing information about Addison's disease and its symptoms, as well as how they can help in the event of an adrenal crisis.

Effective communication with employers and colleagues can also help reduce stress and anxiety in the workplace. By being transparent about your condition and needs, you can alleviate any concerns or misunderstandings that may arise. Remember that your health and well-being are a top priority, and it is okay to ask for help when needed. Overall, open and honest communication is key to successfully navigating the workplace with Addison's disease.

By educating your employer and colleagues, you can create a supportive environment that allows you to thrive in your job while managing your chronic illness effectively. Remember to advocate for yourself and your needs, and don't be afraid to ask for accommodations or support when necessary.

Prioritizing Self-Care in Social Situations

Prioritizing self-care in social situations is crucial for individuals living with Addison's disease. It is important to be mindful of your health needs and limitations when engaging in social activities. By taking proactive steps to care for yourself, you can better manage your condition and enjoy a fulfilling social life.

One key aspect of prioritizing self-care in social situations is managing stress and anxiety. Stress can have a significant impact on your adrenal function, so it is important to find healthy ways to cope with stress. This may include practicing relaxation techniques, engaging in regular exercise, or seeking support from a therapist or support group. By taking steps to manage stress, you can help prevent adrenal crises and maintain your overall well- being.

Nutrition and dietary considerations are also important for individuals with Addison's disease, especially when navigating social situations. It is important to pay attention to your dietary needs and make choices that support your health. This may include avoiding certain foods that can exacerbate your symptoms, such as high- sodium or high-sugar foods, and ensuring that you are getting the nutrients your body needs to function optimally.

When it comes to exercising safely with Addison's disease, it is important to listen to your body and communicate with your healthcare team about your exercise routine. Engaging in regular physical activity can help improve your overall health and well-being, but it is important to find a balance that works for you. By prioritizing safe and appropriate exercise, you can support your adrenal function and maintain your fitness levels.

Balancing work and social life with Addison's disease can be challenging, but it is important to prioritize self-care in order to thrive. This may include setting boundaries, practicing self-compassion, and seeking support from friends, family, or colleagues. By taking proactive steps to care for yourself, you can better manage your condition and enjoy a fulfilling social life.

Setting Boundaries and Managing Expectations

Setting boundaries and managing expectations are essential skills for individuals living with Addison's disease. It is important to recognize your limitations and communicate them effectively to others in order to maintain your health and well-being. By setting boundaries, you can prevent yourself from becoming overwhelmed and reduce the risk of triggering adrenal crises.

Managing expectations is also crucial for those with Addison's disease. It is important to be realistic about what you can and cannot do, and to communicate this to others. By managing expectations, you can avoid unnecessary stress and pressure, which can have a negative impact on your health.

One way to set boundaries and manage expectations is to prioritize self-care. This means taking the time to rest, eat well, and engage in activities that promote physical and emotional well-being. By prioritizing self-care, you can prevent burnout and better manage the symptoms of Addison's disease.

Another important aspect of setting boundaries and managing expectations is communication.

It is important to be open and honest with others about your needs and limitations. By communicating effectively, you can prevent misunderstandings and ensure that others are aware of how they can support you in managing your condition.

Overall, setting boundaries and managing expectations are key components of thriving with Addison's disease. By prioritizing self-care, communicating effectively, and being realistic about your capabilities, you can better manage your condition and live a fulfilling life despite the challenges that come with it.

CHAPTER 7: TRAVELING WITH ADDISON'S

Planning Ahead for Travel

I have always loved to travel and the year without a vacation of some kind has always seemed woefully incomplete to me, as though something vital had been missed. I haven't allowed Addison's to interfere with my vacations and other travel, but to do so safely and comfortably requires a degree of foresight.

Planning ahead for travel is essential for individuals with Addison's, as it necessitates careful consideration and preparation to ensure a safe and enjoyable trip. When traveling with Addison's, it is important to pack all necessary medications, including extra doses in case of unexpected delays or emergencies. It is also recommended to carry a medical alert card or bracelet that indicates your condition, as well as emergency contact information.

In addition to medications, it is crucial to pack snacks and drinks that can help regulate blood sugar levels and prevent adrenal crises (a few 1-ounce cheese nibbles, some almonds and/or a protein bar are good for this purpose).

Planning your meals ahead of time can also help ensure that you are consuming the necessary nutrients to maintain your health while traveling. Avoiding high-fat or high-sodium foods can help prevent complications related to Addison's disease.

When traveling, it is important to have a plan in place for managing stress and anxiety, as these factors can exacerbate symptoms of Addison's. Engaging in relaxation techniques such as deep breathing exercises, meditation, or yoga can help alleviate stress and promote a sense of calm during your trip. It is also helpful to schedule regular breaks and rest periods to prevent fatigue and exhaustion.

Exercising safely while traveling with Addison's disease is possible with proper planning and precautions. It is important to consult with your healthcare provider before engaging in any physical activity, and to listen to your body's signals to avoid overexertion. Low-impact exercises such as walking, swimming, or gentle yoga can help maintain muscle strength and flexibility while traveling.

Overall, planning ahead for travel with Addison's disease involves careful consideration of medication management, dietary needs, stress management, and exercise precautions. By taking proactive steps to prepare for your trip, you can minimize the risk of adrenal crises and ensure a safe and enjoyable travel experience. Remember to reach out to your support system or healthcare provider for guidance and assistance as needed.

Packing Essentials for Trips

As someone who has been diagnosed with Addison's disease, it is important to be prepared when traveling to ensure a safe and enjoyable trip. Packing essentials for trips can make a big difference in managing your condition while away from home. In this subchapter, we will discuss the key items you should always have on hand when traveling with Addison's disease.

First and foremost, it is crucial to pack an ample supply of your medication. Make sure to bring more than enough to last the duration of your trip, as well as extra in case of unexpected delays. It is also a good idea to split your medication between your carry-on bag and checked luggage to prevent any issues in case one gets lost or stolen.

If you think you're going to run out of your medications make arrangements for a pharmacy in the area you're visiting to fill your prescriptions.

In addition to your medication, it is essential to pack snacks and drinks that can help regulate your blood sugar and prevent adrenal crises. Opt for items high in protein and complex carbohydrates, such as nuts, seeds, and whole grain crackers. It is also important to stay hydrated, so be sure to pack a refillable water bottle and drink plenty of fluids throughout your journey.

When traveling with Addison's disease, it is wise to bring a medical alert bracelet or necklace that clearly states your condition. In case of an emergency, this can help medical professionals quickly identify and treat your condition. It is also a good idea to carry a list of your medications, dosages, and any allergies or other medical conditions you may have.

Lastly, consider packing a small first aid kit with items such as bandages, antiseptic wipes, and over-the-counter pain relievers. While traveling can be exciting, it can also be unpredictable, so having these essentials on hand can help you feel more prepared and in control. Remember, taking the time to pack these essentials for trips can make a significant difference in managing your Addison's disease while on the go.

Coping with Changes in Routine

Living with Addison's disease can bring about many challenges, including having to cope with changes in routine. For individuals with this chronic illness, maintaining a consistent daily schedule is crucial in managing symptoms and preventing adrenal crises. However, life is unpredictable, and unexpected events or circumstances can disrupt even the most well-planned routines. In this subchapter, we will explore strategies for coping with changes in routine and adapting to new circumstances while living with Addison's disease.

Managing stress and anxiety is essential for individuals with Addison's disease, as these emotions can exacerbate symptoms and lead to adrenal crises. When faced with changes in routine, it is normal to feel anxious or stressed about how it may impact your health. To cope with these feelings, it is important to practice relaxation techniques such as deep breathing, meditation, or yoga. Additionally, reaching out to a therapist or support group can provide valuable emotional support and coping strategies for managing stress and anxiety related to changes in routine.

Nutrition and dietary considerations play a significant role in managing Addison's disease and adapting to changes in routine. When routines are disrupted, it can be challenging to maintain a healthy diet and eat at regular intervals. To ensure stable blood sugar levels and energy throughout the day, it is essential to plan ahead and have nutritious snacks on hand. Consulting with a dietitian or nutritionist can also help you create a meal plan that accommodates changes in routine while meeting your dietary needs as someone with Addison's disease.

Exercising safely with Addison's disease is another important aspect of coping with changes in routine. Regular physical activity can help manage stress, improve mood, and maintain overall health. However, it is crucial to exercise safely and adjust your workout routine based on changes in your schedule or energy levels. Listening to your body, staying hydrated, and monitoring your symptoms during exercise are key factors in preventing adrenal crises and maintaining a healthy lifestyle with Addison's disease.

Balancing work and social life while living with Addison's disease can be challenging, especially when routine changes occur unexpectedly. Communicating with your employer or colleagues about your condition and any accommodations you may need can help alleviate stress and ensure a supportive work environment. Similarly, maintaining open communication with friends and family about your health needs and limitations can help you navigate social events and activities while managing Addison's disease. Remember that it is okay to prioritize self-care and set boundaries to protect your health and well-being while adapting to changes in routine.

CHAPTER 8: COPING WITH ADRENAL CRISES

Recognizing the Signs of an Adrenal Crisis

I myself have suffered only one adrenal crisis, brought on by a combination of factors: I had just returned from Kentucky to my home in New Jersey, having visited my ex-partner as they were about to enter a hospice, themselves facing the terminal phase of an inoperable cancer.

The stress of travel and the emotional turmoil in the face of their impending death provoked the crisis, but there were warning signs aplenty. My brother- and sister-in-law accompanying me had voiced their concern over my persistent fatigue, nausea, diarrhea, and terrific back pain, but I failed to heed the signs.

Shortly after my return home, the symptoms became so profoundly intense that they couldn't be ignored. Nausea became interminable vomiting, diarrhea became bloody, and fatigue became paralysis. It was when my vision began to blur that I knew steps had to be taken and an ambulance was called. Had that call not been made, I would have died.

The point is that adrenal crises are emergencies. To ignore them is not to court death – to ignore them is to die.

Recognizing the signs of an adrenal crisis is crucial for individuals who have been diagnosed with Addison's disease. An adrenal crisis, also known as an adrenal crisis, can be life-threatening if not promptly treated. It occurs when the body does not have enough cortisol, a hormone produced by the adrenal glands, to manage stress and regulate various bodily functions. By being able to identify the signs of an adrenal crisis, individuals can take immediate action to prevent serious complications.

Some common signs of an adrenal crisis include sudden and severe fatigue, weakness, dizziness, nausea, vomiting, abdominal pain, and confusion. These symptoms may escalate rapidly and can lead to a state of shock if not addressed promptly. It is important for individuals with Addison's disease to be aware of their body's signals and seek medical attention immediately if they suspect they are experiencing an adrenal crisis.

In addition to physical symptoms, emotional and mental changes can also indicate an adrenal crisis. These may include sudden mood swings, irritability, anxiety, and confusion. It is essential for individuals with Addison's disease to pay attention to these changes and not dismiss them as unrelated to their condition. Seeking help from a healthcare provider or loved one during an adrenal crisis is crucial for receiving timely treatment and support.

To effectively manage an adrenal crisis, individuals with Addison's disease should have an emergency plan in place. This plan should include instructions on how to administer emergency injections of cortisol, as well as when to seek medical attention. It is also important to educate family members, friends, and coworkers about the signs of an adrenal crisis and how they can help in case of an emergency. By being prepared and proactive, individuals can reduce the risk of serious complications during an adrenal crisis.

In conclusion, recognizing the signs of an adrenal crisis is essential for individuals living with Addison's disease. By being vigilant and proactive in monitoring their symptoms, individuals can take the necessary steps to prevent a life-threatening emergency. It is important to have an emergency plan in place, educate others about the signs of an adrenal crisis, and seek help immediately if experiencing symptoms. With proper awareness and preparedness, individuals with Addison's disease can effectively manage adrenal crises and live well with their chronic illness.

Emergency Response and Treatment

In the event of an adrenal crisis, it is crucial for individuals with Addison's disease to be prepared and know how to respond effectively. An adrenal crisis is a life- threatening situation that occurs when the body is not producing enough cortisol, which is essential for regulating blood pressure and responding to stress. Symptoms of an adrenal crisis can include severe fatigue, dizziness, nausea, vomiting, and confusion. If you experience these symptoms, it is important to seek emergency medical treatment immediately.

Treatment for an adrenal crisis typically involves receiving intravenous fluids and corticosteroids to restore cortisol levels in the body. It is essential to carry an emergency injection kit with you at all times, containing a syringe with a pre-filled dose of hydrocortisone.

This kit can be a lifesaver in the event of an adrenal crisis, allowing you to quickly administer the necessary medication to prevent serious complications.

In addition to knowing how to respond to an adrenal crisis, it is important to take proactive steps to prevent one from occurring in the first place. This includes regularly monitoring your cortisol levels, following a consistent medication regimen, and avoiding triggers that can lead to stress or illness. By staying vigilant and proactive in managing your condition, you can reduce the risk of experiencing an adrenal crisis and maintain better overall health and well-being.

It is also important to communicate with your healthcare provider about any concerns or questions you may have regarding emergency response and treatment for Addison's disease. Your healthcare team can provide valuable guidance and support in developing a personalized plan for managing adrenal crises and staying safe and healthy.

Remember, you are not alone in this journey, and there are resources and support systems available to help you navigate the challenges of living with Addison's disease.

By being informed, prepared, and proactive in your approach to emergency response and treatment, you can effectively manage your condition and thrive with Addison's disease. Remember to prioritize your health and well-being, and don't hesitate to reach out for help when needed. With the right support and resources, you can lead a fulfilling and healthy life with Addison's disease.

Preventative Measures to Avoid Crises

Living with Addison's disease can present a number of challenges, including the potential for adrenal crises. However, there are steps you can take to help prevent crises from occurring. One of the most important preventative measures is to always carry an emergency kit with you that includes extra medication, a list of your medications and dosages, and information on how to administer an emergency injection of cortisol. This kit can be a lifesaver in the event of a crisis, so be sure to keep it with you at all times.

Managing stress and anxiety is also crucial in preventing adrenal crises. Stress can trigger a crisis by putting strain on your body's already compromised adrenal glands. It's important to find healthy ways to cope with stress, such as practicing relaxation techniques like deep breathing, meditation, or yoga. Additionally, seeking support from a therapist or support group can help you manage anxiety and stress more effectively.

Nutrition and dietary considerations play a key role in preventing adrenal crises as well. It's important to maintain a balanced diet that includes plenty of fruits, vegetables, whole grains, and lean proteins. Avoiding high- sugar and high-sodium foods can help regulate your blood sugar levels and prevent spikes that could trigger a crisis. Be sure to also stay hydrated and monitor your electrolyte levels to support your adrenal health.

Exercising safely with Addison's disease is another important preventative measure. While exercise is beneficial for overall health, it's important to listen to your body and not push yourself too hard. Be sure to monitor your energy levels and adjust your exercise routine as needed. It's also important to stay hydrated and replenish electrolytes during and after exercise to prevent a crisis.

Balancing work and social life with Addison's disease can be challenging, but it's important to prioritize self-care and stress management to prevent crises. Be sure to communicate your needs with your employer and colleagues, and don't be afraid to ask for accommodations if needed. It's also important to maintain a healthy work-life balance and prioritize relaxation and self-care activities to prevent burnout. By taking these preventative measures, you can reduce your risk of adrenal crises and thrive with Addison's disease.

CHAPTER 9: SUPPORT SYSTEMS AND RESOURCES FOR INDIVIDUALS WITH ADDISON'S

Online Communities and Support Groups

I mentioned the old song above, *"You've got to have friends!"* When I was first diagnosed, being an enthusiastic Facebook user, I made a beeline to look for any pertinent online groups I could find. My search was rewarded with a number of excellent Facebook forums in which Addison's patients can find mutual support and exchange notes, news and tips, hints, and observations.

Some examples include Living with Addison's Disease (13k members), Addison's Disease Adrenal Sufficiency – One Day at a Time (8.1k members), Addison's Disease Support and Self-Help Group (5.2k members), Addison's Disease Awareness Group (3.7k members) and a few others.

These have the advantage of having amongst their members individuals who have battled Addison's for a long time, have much experience in dealing with its demands, and can offer valuable technical (albeit not medical) and emotional support. Because Addison's is a rare disorder it is unlikely one would have a family member or acquaintance close at hand who is also diagnosed.

Online communities and support groups can be invaluable resources for individuals who have been diagnosed with Addison's disease. These virtual spaces provide a platform for connecting with others who are also living with the condition, offering a sense of community and understanding that can be difficult to find in everyday life. Through these online communities, individuals can share their experiences, ask questions, and offer support to one another.

Living with Addison's disease can be challenging, and managing stress and anxiety is an important aspect of maintaining overall health and well-being. Online support groups can provide a safe space for individuals to discuss their feelings and concerns, as well as learn coping strategies from others who are facing similar challenges. By connecting with others who understand the unique struggles of living with Addison's, individuals can feel less alone and more supported in their journey.

Nutrition and dietary considerations play a crucial role in managing Addison's disease, as certain foods and beverages can impact cortisol levels and overall health. Online communities and support groups often provide valuable information and resources on how to eat a balanced diet that supports adrenal function. By connecting with others who have experience with managing their diet and nutrition, individuals with Addison's can gain insight and practical tips for making healthy food choices.

Exercising safely with Addison's disease is another important aspect of managing the condition. Online support groups can be a great resource for individuals looking to incorporate physical activity into their routine while taking into consideration the challenges of living with adrenal insufficiency. By sharing experiences and advice on how to exercise safely, members of these communities can help each other stay active and maintain their overall health.

In addition to providing practical information and resources, online communities and support groups can also offer emotional support and encouragement to individuals with Addison's disease. Coping with adrenal crises, balancing work and social life, traveling, parenting, and navigating relationships can all be complex and challenging tasks for those living with a chronic illness. By connecting with others who are facing similar challenges, individuals can find comfort, advice, and understanding in these virtual communities. Through the support of these online networks, individuals with Addison's can feel empowered to navigate the ups and downs of life with chronic illness.

Accessing Healthcare and Insurance Resources

Accessing healthcare and insurance resources is a crucial aspect of managing Addison's disease effectively. As a chronic illness, Addison's requires ongoing medical care and monitoring to ensure that symptoms are managed and potential complications are addressed promptly. It is important for individuals with Addison's to have access to healthcare providers who are knowledgeable about the condition and who can provide comprehensive care.

Health insurance coverage is essential for individuals with Addison's, as the costs of medications, doctor's visits, and emergency care can add up quickly. It is important for individuals with Addison's to understand their insurance coverage and to know what services are covered under their plan.

This may involve working closely with insurance providers to ensure that necessary medications and treatments are covered and that out-of-pocket costs are minimized.

In addition to healthcare and insurance resources, individuals with Addison's may benefit from support systems and resources that can help them navigate the challenges of living with a chronic illness. Support groups, online forums, and advocacy organizations can provide valuable information and emotional support for individuals with Addison's. These resources can also help individuals connect with others who are facing similar challenges and share strategies for managing their condition effectively.

When traveling with Addison's, it is important to plan ahead and ensure that necessary medications and supplies are readily available.

This may involve carrying a medical alert card or bracelet, as well as a written care plan that outlines specific instructions for managing an adrenal crisis. It is also important to research healthcare facilities at your destination and to have a plan in place for accessing medical care if needed.

Overall, accessing healthcare and insurance resources is an essential part of managing Addison's disease effectively.

By staying informed about insurance coverage, connecting with support resources, and planning ahead for travel and emergencies, individuals with Addison's can take control of their health and well-being and thrive despite the challenges of living with a chronic illness.

Counseling and Therapy Services

Counseling and therapy services can be invaluable resources for individuals living with Addison's disease. The emotional toll of managing a chronic illness can be significant, and having a professional to talk to can help individuals cope with the stress and anxiety that often accompany a diagnosis of Addison's. Counseling can provide a safe space to explore feelings of fear, frustration, and sadness, as well as develop coping strategies for managing these emotions.

Therapy services can also be beneficial for individuals with Addison's who may be struggling to navigate the challenges of balancing work and social life while managing their condition. A therapist can help individuals set boundaries, prioritize self-care, and communicate effectively with employers, friends, and family members about their needs. Additionally, therapy can be a valuable tool for addressing any mental health concerns that may arise as a result of living with a chronic illness.

Nutrition and dietary considerations are essential aspects of managing Addison's disease, and therapy services can provide guidance on creating a balanced and nourishing diet that supports overall health and well-being. A therapist can help individuals develop a healthy relationship with food, navigate food restrictions, and address any emotional eating patterns that may be impacting their health.

Exercising safely with Addison's is another important aspect of managing the condition, and therapy services can offer support and guidance on developing an appropriate exercise routine that is tailored to individual needs and abilities. A therapist can help individuals set realistic fitness goals, address any fears or concerns about exercising with Addison's, and develop strategies for staying motivated and consistent with their exercise regimen.

Indeed, counseling and therapy services can be valuable tools for individuals living with Addison's disease to support their mental and emotional well-being, navigate the complexities of managing their condition, and improve their overall quality of life. By seeking out these services, individuals with Addison's can build a strong support system, develop effective coping strategies, and cultivate resilience in the face of the challenges that come with living with a chronic illness.

CHAPTER 10: PARENTING WITH ADDISON'S

Managing Parenthood Responsibilities with a Chronic Illness

Anyone who is a frequent airline passenger must know the ritual words of the flight attendant invariably offered before takeoff: *"In the event of a drop in cabin pressure, an emergency mask with oxygen will drop from the ceiling above your seat. Follow the instructions printed on your passenger card and affix your own mask before attempting to help anyone else."*

Sound advice for airline passengers, and very sound – in fact indispensable - advice for parents with Addison's.

Parenthood is a challenging and rewarding experience for anyone, but when you have been diagnosed with a demanding chronic illness such as Addison's disease, managing the responsibilities of parenthood can become even more complex. In this subchapter, we will explore some strategies and tips for managing parenthood responsibilities while living with Addison's disease.

One of the most important aspects of managing parenthood with a chronic illness is prioritizing self-care.

As a parent with Addison's disease, it is crucial to take care of your own health and well-being in order to be able to care for your children effectively. This may involve setting boundaries, asking for help when needed, and making time for rest and relaxation.

Stress and anxiety can exacerbate symptoms of Addison's disease, so it is important to find healthy ways to manage these emotions. This may include practicing mindfulness and relaxation techniques, seeking support from a therapist or support group, and finding ways to reduce stress in your daily life. By taking care of your mental health, you can better cope with the challenges of parenthood and chronic illness.

Nutrition and dietary considerations play a crucial role in managing Addison's disease, especially for parents who need to maintain energy levels to keep up with their children. It is important to work with a healthcare provider or nutritionist to develop a balanced and nutritious meal plan that meets your individual needs. This may include monitoring your sodium intake, staying hydrated, and eating regular, well-balanced meals.

Exercising safely with Addison's disease is also important for overall health and well-being. While physical activity is beneficial, it is important to listen to your body and avoid overexertion. Consult with your healthcare provider to develop an exercise plan that is safe and appropriate for your condition. By staying active, you can improve your physical and mental health, which can benefit both you and your children.

Balancing work and social life with parenting and a chronic illness can be challenging, but it is possible with careful planning and support. Communicate openly with your employer about your health needs and consider flexible work options if necessary. Lean on your support system of family and friends for help with childcare and household tasks. By prioritizing self-care, managing stress, and seeking support, you can navigate the demands of parenthood with Addison's disease more effectively.

Communicating with Children about Addison's Disease

Communicating with children about Addison's Disease is an

important aspect of managing the condition as a parent or guardian. It is essential to educate children about what Addison's Disease is, how it affects the body, and what to do in case of an emergency. By providing age-appropriate information, children can better understand and support their loved ones with Addison's Disease.

When communicating with children about Addison's Disease, it is crucial to use simple language and avoid overwhelming them with too much information at once. Start by explaining that Addison's Disease is a chronic illness that affects the adrenal glands, which are responsible for producing hormones that help the body respond to stress. Let them know that people with Addison's Disease may need to take medication daily and be mindful of their stress levels.

It is also important to reassure children that Addison's Disease is manageable with proper medication and lifestyle adjustments. Encourage open communication and answer any questions they may have about the condition. By fostering a supportive and understanding environment, children can feel more comfortable and confident in supporting their family member with Addison's Disease.

In addition to explaining the basics of Addison's Disease to children, it is essential to teach them how to recognize and respond to adrenal crises. Make sure they know the signs and symptoms of an adrenal crisis, such as severe fatigue, nausea, vomiting, and dizziness, and what steps to take in case of an emergency. Practice emergency scenarios with them to ensure they are prepared to act quickly and seek help if needed.

Communicating with children about Addison's Disease is a crucial part of managing the condition as a family. By educating children about the illness, providing support, and teaching them how to respond in emergencies, you can help them feel empowered and knowledgeable about how to support their loved one with Addison's Disease. Remember to approach the topic with sensitivity and patience, and encourage open dialogue to ensure children feel informed and supported.

Seeking Support from Family and Friends

Living with Addison's disease can be challenging, but having a strong support system in place can make a world of difference. Seeking support from family and friends is crucial in managing the physical and emotional aspects of this chronic illness. It is important to communicate openly with your loved ones about your condition and how it affects your daily life. By educating them about Addison's disease, you can help them better understand your needs and provide the support you require.

Managing stress and anxiety is essential for individuals with Addison's disease, as these factors can exacerbate symptoms and lead to adrenal crises. Seeking support from family and friends can help in reducing stress levels and providing emotional support during difficult times. By sharing your feelings and concerns with loved ones, you can receive the comfort and reassurance you need to cope with the challenges of living with a chronic illness.

Nutrition and dietary considerations play a significant role in managing Addison's disease. It is important to follow a balanced diet that includes sufficient amounts of sodium and potassium to support adrenal function. Seeking support from family and friends can make meal planning easier and ensure that you are meeting your nutritional needs. By involving your loved ones in your dietary choices, you can create a supportive environment that promotes healthy eating habits.

Exercising safely with Addison's disease requires careful planning and monitoring of your physical activity. Seeking support from family and friends can help you stay motivated and accountable in maintaining a regular exercise routine. By involving your loved ones in your fitness goals, you can receive encouragement and assistance in staying active while managing your symptoms effectively

Balancing work and social life with Addison's disease can be challenging, but having a strong support system can help you navigate these complexities. Seeking support from family and friends can provide you with the emotional support and practical assistance you need to manage your responsibilities effectively. By communicating your needs and limitations with your loved ones, you can create a supportive network that enables you to thrive in both your professional and personal life.

CHAPTER 11: MENTAL HEALTH AND SELF-CARE FOR THOSE WITH ADDISON'S

Importance of Mental Health in Managing Addison's

Chronic illnesses are like the uninvited guest who never seems to want to leave. They stick around, unbidden, sometimes for a lifetime, reshaping the way our bodies function and our minds work. Addison's disease is just one example of a number of these unrelenting and burdensome companions.

Living with Addison's disease presents some unique challenges, both physically and mentally. One important aspect of managing this chronic illness is prioritizing mental health. Mental health plays a crucial role in overall well-being and can greatly impact how individuals cope with the daily demands of living with Addison's. By focusing on mental health, individuals can better manage stress, anxiety, and other emotional challenges that may arise.

Managing stress and anxiety is particularly important for individuals with Addison's disease, as these conditions can exacerbate symptoms and lead to adrenal crises. By practicing stress-reducing techniques such as mindfulness, meditation, yoga and deep breathing exercises, individuals can better regulate their cortisol levels and prevent potential health complications. Additionally, seeking therapy or counseling can provide valuable support in managing anxiety and improving overall mental health.

Nutrition and dietary considerations are also essential in managing Addison's disease and promoting mental well-being. A balanced diet rich in nutrient-dense foods can help regulate blood sugar levels, support adrenal function, and improve mood and energy levels. Avoiding foods high in sugar, caffeine, and processed ingredients can help stabilize cortisol levels and prevent mood swings and fatigue.

Exercising safely with Addison's disease is another key component of maintaining mental health. Regular physical activity can help reduce stress, boost mood, and improve overall well-being. However, individuals with Addison's should exercise caution and consult with their healthcare provider before starting a new exercise routine to ensure it is safe and appropriate for their specific needs.

In addition to managing physical symptoms, individuals with Addison's must also prioritize self-care and mental well-being. This may include setting boundaries, practicing self-compassion, seeking support from loved ones, and engaging in activities that bring joy and relaxation. By prioritizing mental health and self-care, individuals can better navigate the challenges of living with Addison's disease and lead fulfilling and balanced lives.

Self-Care Practices for Emotional Well- Being

Go easy on yourself – whatever you manage to do today, let it be enough.

Self-care practices are essential for maintaining emotional well-being while living with Addison's disease. Managing stress and anxiety is particularly important for individuals with this chronic illness, as stress can exacerbate symptoms and lead to adrenal crises. It is important to prioritize self-care activities that promote relaxation and reduce stress, such as meditation, deep breathing exercises, and gentle yoga practices. Taking time for yourself and engaging in activities that bring you joy can help to improve your overall emotional well-being.

Nutrition and dietary considerations are also crucial for individuals with Addison's disease. Maintaining a balanced diet that includes plenty of fruits, vegetables, whole grains, and lean proteins can help to support adrenal function and overall health. It is important to eat regular meals and snacks throughout the day to help stabilize blood sugar levels and prevent hypoglycemia. Avoiding processed foods, caffeine, and alcohol can also help to reduce stress on the body and support adrenal health.

Exercising safely with Addison's disease is possible, but it is important to listen to your body and adjust your workout routine accordingly. Low-impact exercises such as walking, swimming, and yoga can be beneficial for individuals with this chronic illness. It is important to stay hydrated, take breaks when needed, and monitor your symptoms during exercise. Consulting with a healthcare provider or a physical therapist can help you develop a safe and effective exercise plan.

Balancing work, family and social life with Addison's disease can be challenging, but it is important to prioritize self-care and set boundaries to prevent burnout. Communicating with your employer and coworkers about your condition can help to create a supportive work environment. Making time for social activities and connecting with friends and loved ones can also help to improve your emotional well-being and reduce feelings of isolation.

In conclusion, self-care practices are essential for individuals living with Addison's disease. By making priorities of stress management, nutrition, exercise, and self-care activities, you can effectively manage your symptoms and improve your quality of life. Remember to listen to your body, seek support from healthcare providers and loved ones, and take time for yourself to rest and recharge.

Seeking Professional Help

Seeking professional help for mental health concerns is an important aspect of managing Addison's disease. It is common for individuals with chronic illnesses like Addison's to experience feelings of anxiety, stress, and depression. These mental health concerns can have a significant impact on overall well-being and can even exacerbate physical symptoms of the disease. Seeking support from a mental health professional, such as a therapist or counselor, can provide valuable tools and strategies for coping with these challenges.

When seeking professional help for mental health concerns, it is important to find a provider who is knowledgeable about Addison's disease and its unique challenges. A mental health professional who understands the physical and emotional aspects of living with a chronic illness like Addison's can provide more effective support and guidance. It may be helpful to seek out a therapist who has experience working with individuals with chronic illnesses or who specializes in treating anxiety and stress.

In addition to therapy, medication may also be a helpful tool in managing mental health concerns related to Addison's disease. Some individuals with Addison's may benefit from medications such as antidepressants or anti- anxiety medications to help alleviate symptoms of depression and anxiety. It is important to work closely with a healthcare provider to find the right medication and dosage that works best for you.

Support groups can also be a valuable resource for individuals with Addison's disease who are seeking professional help for mental health concerns. Connecting with others who understand the challenges of living with a chronic illness can provide a sense of community and validation. Support groups can offer a safe space to share experiences, gain insight, and receive encouragement from others who are on a similar journey.

Overall, seeking professional help for mental health concerns is an important part of managing Addison's disease. By working with a mental health professional who understands the unique challenges of living with a chronic illness, individuals with Addison's can develop effective strategies for coping with anxiety, stress, and depression. Whether through therapy, medication, support groups, or a combination of these resources, seeking help for mental health concerns can lead to improved well-being and a better quality of life.

CHAPTER 12: NAVIGATING RELATIONSHIPS AND DATING WITH ADDISON'S

Communicating about Addison's Disease with Loved Ones

Addison's disease might hide the person underneath, but there's still a person there who needs your love and attention. Being deeply loved by someone gives you strength while loving someone deeply gives you courage. Don't believe that caring deeply and being cared for cannot change our lives. Indeed, a few caring people can change the world.

Communicating about your Addison's disease with loved ones is an important aspect of managing this chronic illness. It can be challenging to explain the complexities of Addison's to family and friends, but open and honest communication is key to receiving the support you need. By educating your loved ones about Addison's disease, you can help them better understand your condition and how it affects your daily life.

When discussing your Addison's disease with loved ones, it's important to be clear and concise in your communication. Provide them with basic information about the condition, such as how it affects the adrenal glands and the importance of taking medication regularly. You may also want to explain common symptoms of Addison's, such as fatigue, muscle weakness, and low blood pressure, so that your loved ones can recognize when you may be experiencing a flare-up.

It's also important to communicate your needs and limitations to your loved ones. Let them know how Addison's disease impacts your daily routine and what accommodations or support you may need. By being open about your needs, you can ensure that your loved ones are able to provide the necessary assistance and understanding.

In addition to educating your loved ones about Addison's disease, it's important to communicate your feelings and emotions with them. Living with a chronic illness can be emotionally challenging, and it's important to have a support system in place. By sharing your thoughts and feelings with your loved ones, you can receive the emotional support you need to cope with the challenges of Addison's disease.

Communicating about Addison's disease with loved ones is essential for managing this chronic illness effectively. By educating your family and friends, expressing your needs and limitations, and sharing your emotions, you can build a strong support system that will help you thrive with Addison's disease. Remember that you are not alone in this journey, and your loved ones are there to support you every step of the way.

Dating Tips and Strategies for Disclosure

Dating can be a daunting experience for anyone, but for those with Addison's disease, there may be additional challenges to navigate.

When it comes to disclosing your condition to a potential partner, it's important to approach the conversation with honesty and confidence. One tip is to choose an appropriate time and place to have this conversation, where you feel comfortable and have the space to explain your condition fully. It's also helpful to have resources on hand to provide your partner with more information about Addison's disease, so they can better understand how it may impact your relationship.

When discussing your Addison's disease with a potential

partner, it's essential to focus on the positive aspects of how you manage your condition rather than dwelling on the potential challenges. Highlight the ways in which you take care of yourself, such as monitoring your medication, eating a balanced diet, and managing stress effectively. This can help reassure your partner that you are proactive about your health and that you are capable of maintaining a fulfilling relationship despite your chronic illness.

In terms of strategies for disclosure, it may be helpful to practice what you want to say beforehand so that you feel confident and prepared when the conversation arises. Be prepared for questions from your partner and try to answer them openly and honestly.

Remember that communication is key in any relationship, and being transparent about your Addison's disease can help build trust and understanding between you and your partner.

It's also important to remember that not everyone will react the same way to your disclosure. Some people may be more understanding and accepting, while others may struggle to come to terms with your chronic illness. It's essential to be patient and give your partner time to process the information and ask any questions they may have. Ultimately, dating with Addison's disease is about finding someone who accepts and supports you for who you are, including your health condition.

Navigating relationships and dating with Addison's disease may require some additional thought and effort, but it is entirely possible to find love and companionship while managing your chronic illness. By approaching the conversation with honesty and positivity, focusing on self- care and communication, and being patient with your partner's reactions, you can build strong and fulfilling relationships that support your well-being and happiness.

Building Healthy Relationships while Managing a ChronicIllness

Building healthy relationships while managing a chronic illness like Addison's disease can be challenging, but it is essential for overall well-being. Communication is key in any relationship, especially when it comes to discussing your illness with loved ones. Be open and honest about your needs and limitations, and educate them about Addison's disease so they can better understand how to support you.

Living with Addison's disease can be overwhelming at times, and it is important to prioritize self-care and manage stress and anxiety effectively. Practice relaxation techniques such as deep breathing, meditation, or yoga to help calm your mind and body. Seeking therapy or counseling can also be beneficial in learning coping strategies and building resilience in the face of chronic illness.

It cannot be overemphasized that nutrition plays a crucial role in managing Addison's disease, as certain foods can impact cortisol levels. It is important to maintain a balanced diet rich in fruits, vegetables, whole grains, and lean proteins. Avoiding processed foods, excessive caffeine, and alcohol can help stabilize blood sugar levels and support adrenal function. Consulting with a registered dietitian can provide personalized guidance on dietary considerations for individuals with Addison's.

Exercising safely with Addison's disease is possible with proper planning and monitoring. Start with low-impact activities like walking, swimming, or yoga, and gradually increase intensity as tolerated. Be mindful of your energy levels and listen to your body's cues to prevent overexertion. Always carry emergency medication, such as a cortisol injection, when engaging in physical activity to prevent adrenal crises.

Balancing work and social life with Addison's disease may require adjustments to accommodate your health needs. Communicate with your employer about any accommodations or flexibility needed to manage your condition effectively. Prioritize self-care and set boundaries to prevent burnout. Lean on your support system, whether it be family, friends, or online communities, for encouragement and understanding as you navigate life with Addison's.

FAMOUS PEOPLE WITH ADDISON'S DISEASE

Some famous people who have/had Addison's disease are:

Thomas Addison, British physician after whom the disease is named

Sabino Arana, Basque writer and hero of Basque culture and language; founder of Basque nationalist movement

Jane Austen, Renowned English novelist

Charles Ruijs de Beerenbrouck, Governor of Limburg Province and Netherlands Prime Minister

Elisabeth Catez (Saint Elizabeth of the Trinity) French Roman Catholic Carmelite nun and spiritual writer; died at age 26 of Addison's, canonized a saint in 2016

Andrew Dasburg, American modernist painter

Lawrence Durrell, renowned British novelist and author of the *Alexandria Quartet*

Chris Jackson, Actor and singer best known for his portrayal of George Washington in the musical "Hamilton"

Thomas Story Kirkbride, Influential 19th-century psychiatrist known for his advocacy of humane treatment of the mentally ill

John F. Kennedy, Former president of the United States

Osama bin Laden, Founder of al-Qaeda

Kodi Taehyun Lee, Blind, autistic singer-songwriter and piano savant

Helen Reddy, Australian singer and human rights activist

Eugene Shoemaker, American geologist and one of the founders of Planetary Science

Eunice Kennedy Shriver, Sister of JFK and philanthropist

George Summerbee, English professional footballer

RESOURCES FOR INFORMATION & SUPPORT

NADF: National Adrenal Disease Foundation
www.nadf.us
Telephone: (847) 726-9010
Email:nadfsupport@nadf.us

American Adrenal Association
www.americanadrenals.org
Email: info@americanadrenals.org

The EPIC Foundation
www.epictogether.org
Telephone: (888) 862-5554 Email:
admin@epictogether.org

Adrenal Insufficiency United
www.aiunited.org
Telephone: 503-298-4291 Email: contact@aiunited.org

National Organization for Rare Disorders
www.rarediseases.org
Telephone: (617) 249-7300

The Endocrine Society
www.endocrine.org
Telephone: (202) 736-9705

The American Association of Clinical Endocrinologists
www.aace.com
Telephone: (904) 353-7878 Email: info@aace.com

The Canadian Addison's Disease Society
www.addisonsociety.ca
(888)550-5582   Email: info@addisonsociety.ca